Gluten: The Insidious Protein
A Personal Journey

Copyright Information

Copyright © 2016 by John H. Pope

Paperback ISBN-13: 978-0998300801

E-Book ISBN-13: 978-0998300818

Publisher: John H. Pope

Author: John H. Pope

Title: Gluten: The Insidious Protein (A Personal Journey)

First Edition

Websites

MyGlutenJourney.com

JohnHPope.com

Cover Design: John Pope

Contents

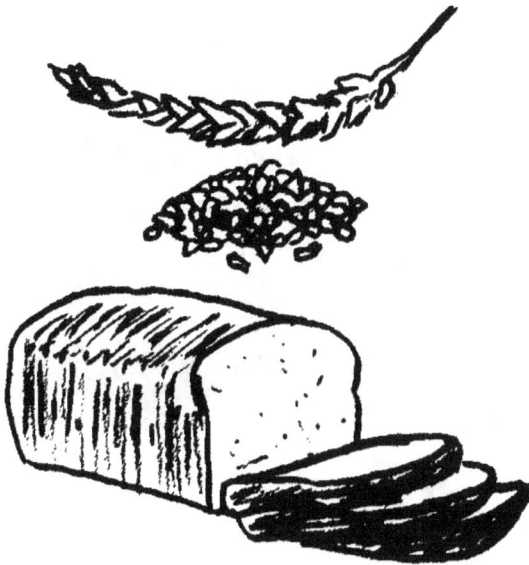

Chapter 1
What is gluten anyway?

Gluten is a protein that is found in wheat, barley, and rye, and it has been around for a long, long time. It is like a glue that helps food keep its shape. Bread would not be fluffy and held together so well if not for gluten. Crumbly pastries that hold the delicious filling would not be so pleasurable when chewed if not for gluten. That is why it is used in so many recipes.

I remember my days when I was eating gluten products. They were delicious! At the time, I completely took them for granted. A pastry with wheat is entirely different than a pastry with some other flour like potato flour, rice flour, or corn flour. The wheat has a consistency that is extremely difficult to mimic with other flours. I have tried many different types of flours, and I have yet to find one that imitates the consistency of wheat. The flours usually produce hard pastries, bread, and crackers, and they have harsh flavors. If they do manage to get the product soft, gluten free products will break apart very easily. And that is precisely why a gluten free diet is so difficult to maintain.

Why Is Gluten Suddenly a Problem?

But why is gluten suddenly such a big health issue? If gluten has been around for thousands of years, why is it, that in the last 50 years or so, there is suddenly a large portion of the population that apparently has some kind of symptoms related to gluten? According to Grainstorm Heritage Baking[i], the answer may lie in the manufacturing process of wheat, barley, and rye.

In ancient times, and actually as near as the industrial revolution in the 1800's, wheat was ground with a stone grinding wheel. It was a relatively long process and the entire wheat kernel was mashed up and used for flour. This flour was very nutritious because the entire kernel was used. However, the portion of the kernel that is not the pure white flour does not keep very well. If the flour is stored for any amount of time, it would go bad. The white flour could be extracted, but only in very small amounts. Thus, only high society and very wealthy people could afford to get it.

During the industrial revolution, a new method of milling the wheat with a steel roller mill was invented and put into mass production. This method shaves off the nutritious part of the wheat kernel and salvages the pure white flour portion of the kernel. This flour is very appealing because it was considered the best part of the kernel. For baking, it is the best part, because this white flour has all of the desirable characteristics for pleasant looking, feeling, and tasting baked goods.

Now we have dozens of products that we can buy off the shelf to bake at home in our own ovens. They will remain usable for months with no fear of pests or spoilage. This revolutionary way of processing wheat put the highly desirable white flour into the hands of everyone. Now a poor family could bake bread just like a high class family. Of course, the biggest problem that no one ever knew at the time, is that the part of the kernel that is shaved off is where all of the nutrients are. So by making this beautiful white flour, the process has accidentally turned wheat, which nourished man for thousands of years, into a lump of white stuff, loaded with gluten and with the nutrition of cardboard.

Another possible contributor to the gluten epidemic is the advent of genetic engineering. When we talk about genetic engineering, what usually comes to mind is a man in a white lab coat injecting the guts of a frog into dinosaur DNA. But genetic engineering can also be as simple as observing characteristics that you would like to see in a plant or animal, and then only breeding or pollenating those plants or animals that have the characteristics of interest. This was done with wheat and many other plants and animals.

Animals you say? That's barbaric! ... But in reality, just think dogs. Why are there so many breeds and why do they all have such outstanding individual characteristics? Why is a beagle a beagle? Why does a Doberman Pincer look the way it does and a poodle look like a poodle? Of course, it is genetic engineering before the term even existed. Humans became aware that, by breeding dogs together with special traits that the humans liked, they could ultimately, over many dog generations, create a new breed. This breed would have its own unique characteristics completely different than any other breeds.

So how does this play into gluten issues you ask? When "modern" wheat was created in the 1900's, all that mattered was how much yield you could get and how well it baked. So what we wound up with was a super wheat that is impervious to pests and grows easily in large fields with high yields, and can be processed into the beautiful white flour that we use today. Again, the problem is that the nutritional value that we get from flour today is practically zero. And, demonstrably, the gluten in this flour is causing many health issues for many different people.

Symptoms of Gluten Intolerance

The potential symptoms of gluten intolerance is quite long. Gluten sufferers can experience one of the symptoms or, as in my case, many of the symptoms. Here is a very incomplete list of symptoms that I have compiled over the years based on my own experiences as well as contributions from other sufferers of gluten intolerance. I have bold faced the symptoms that I had. There are twelve on this list (in bold) that I personally had!

- Abdominal Pain
- Abdominal Cramping
- **Acid Reflux**
- **Bloating**
- **Brittle Nails**
- **Constipation**
- **Depression**
- Dry Hair
- Diarrhea
- **Fatigue/Lethargy**
- Hair Loss (Alopecia)
- **Headaches and Migraines**
- **IBS (Irritable Bowel Syndrome)**
- Joint pain
- **Lactose intolerance**
- **Nausea**
- Numbness or tingling in hands or feet
- **Skin Rash**
- **Vomiting**
- Unexplained Weight loss

Like me when I first became aware, you might be saying to yourself as you look at this list, "I have that... I have that..." I look at the list now, and I still can't believe that I experienced all of those symptoms on a regular basis. It was just part of life, and I became accustomed to it. But I didn't have to become accustomed to it. I can simply change what I eat and make most or all of the symptoms disappear.

The question is of course, "Is gluten causing *your* health issues?"

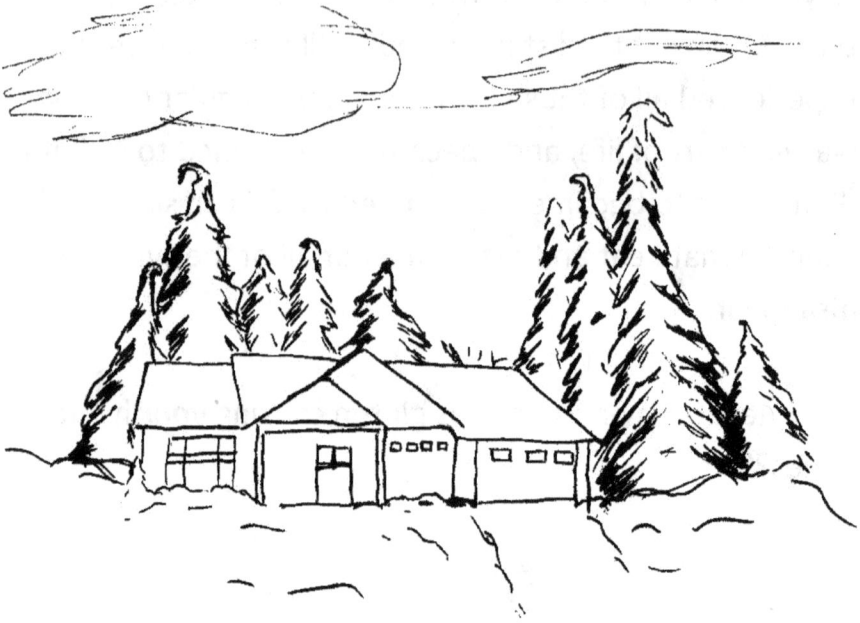

Chapter 2
My Life

30 Years of Misery

Imagine a life where you feel tired all of the time. No matter what you do, or how healthy you try to eat, you just always feel lethargic and run down. Imagine having three migraines a week; having headaches with all of the horrible feelings associated with a real migraine. Wanting nothing but sleep. A quiet dark room to remove yourself from the agony of light and noise. The fear of eating anything because you are afraid it won't stay down, and... the headaches. The intense, throbbing headaches that prevent you from doing things with your friends and family. The ones that cause you to seclude yourself into a dark room and sleep. Not eight hours of sleep like normal people, but sleep of thirteen to twenty hours straight because your body is craving it. Imagine being constipated for days or weeks at a time, and constantly having digestive trouble. Forever rearranging your diet to attempt to feel just a little bit better. Imagine having constant acid reflux or heartburn. Taking antacid constantly, and not being able to pinpoint it to any one food. Imagine seeing doctors... many different doctors: general practitioners, neurologists, allergy, and ear, nose, and throat doctors. All with no resolution or relief to your symptoms. Imagine most of your family just telling you it is stress or it is in your head. Unfortunately, no one else can truly empathize without actually having it happen to them, and no one can sympathize because it just sounds too incredible. How can one person have so many different problems that doctors can't treat? They believe that it must be psychological. If you can imagine all of these things, all happening at the same time, all to one person, then you can imagine what my life was like before I became gluten free.

I call gluten insidious because of the range and seemingly unrelated symptoms that it can cause. My own personal experiences of symptoms, as well as my general observations of people around me, have led me to believe that gluten is probably causing many people a lot of distress in their own lives without them ever knowing or even suspecting what the root cause is.

Let me be clear that I am not a doctor, and I do not have any medical training. This book is my own personal journey of discovery. I have seen many doctors and specialists before I discovered I was gluten intolerant. In the end, it was not my own doctors or specialists at all that diagnosed me. I will get more into that subject in Chapter 3. For now, let's discuss doctors for a moment.

I want everyone to understand that I am not trying to criticize doctors in a negative way. I am only outlining my personal experiences that have led me to where I am today with my own knowledge of gluten intolerance. Modern medicine is definitely a wonder and can do many things to save lives as well as help with quality of life. The medicines that are available can do wondrous things. However, sometimes (maybe many times), the doctors get caught up in the medicines themselves. They become very "Westernized" in the respect that they attempt to treat symptoms rather than find actual root causes. This is not something that I have researched, but rather is gleaned from my personal experiences. Let me give you a few of my personal examples.

Personal Case 1

Along with my gluten issues, I also am unfortunate enough to have been plagued by asthma and allergies when I was younger. When I was about twenty-eight years old, I started coughing a lot. I had just started a new job and I felt pretty good, but I just couldn't stop coughing. We had a company meeting, and during a relatively silent point where the company vice president was speaking, I began coughing.. and coughing.. and coughing. I just couldn't stop. Finally I had to leave the room. I drank some water and I seemed to feel ok and thought nothing more of it.

The following Saturday, I started having a lot of difficulty breathing. My breathing became extremely labored. I tried my usual asthma rescue inhaler, but it had no effect. I decided that maybe I better go to the emergency room. This was before the days that the emergency room treated asthma and breathing disorders as actual emergencies. So when I arrived, I signed in and waited for my turn to be examined by the attending physician.

When I went into the examination room, the first thing they did, which was standard operating procedure at the time, was to give me a breathing treatment. I was no stranger to this having experienced it many times. I inhaled and exhaled the medicine until it was gone. My breathing got better as it usually does, but I could sense that this was not the same as a typical asthma attack. The feeling of being out of breath was more distressed and a little painful, which was not typical.

I sat on the hospital bed and waited the standard wait time of about twenty minutes when the doctor finally showed up. The doctor shook my hand, we exchanged the usual pleasantries, and then he listened to my breathing. He said everything sounded great and that I should be all set to leave. I explained my issues with coughing and how I felt that this asthma attack felt a lot different than a typical one for me. He listened to me caringly and then sent me for an x-ray.

Back to waiting. As everyone knows, in the hospital emergency room it is an endless cycle of waiting rooms. Sign in... wait... see the nurse... wait... see the doctor, go for a test... wait... back to the room... wait... see the doctor... wait... see the nurse... go home. It's a fairly standard operating procedure. I know there are reasons and I get that, but that doesn't make it any less uncomfortable, especially when you really are sick and worried. So there I sat until I was finally called to have my chest x-rays taken. Back to the examination room for some more waiting.

The doctor came in after viewing my x-rays and declared that I have walking pneumonia. He said he could admit me, but that we could probably just treat it at home. In my younger days, I was much less vocal than I am now. Even though in the back of my mind I was thinking that I should definitely be admitted, I meekly nodded my head in agreement. After another brief wait, the nurse came in with my instructions and a prescription. I grabbed my prescription paper, and went home.

I was home for less than an hour when my breathing became labored again. It happened relatively quickly and I became very worried because a breathing treatment usually lasted days for a regular asthma attack. I immediately went back to the emergency room. I walked up to the receptionist and she said, "Can I help you?"... To which I replied "uh... uh... uh..."

I tried talking but nothing would come out, or go in for that matter. I seemed to have lost the ability to breathe. At that point everything is a blur. I remember the receptionist calling out for help. I remember several nurses coming out and practically carrying me into one of the examination rooms. I remember a shot, and nurses all speaking softly trying to calm me down. I remember a tear streaming down my eye. I thought I was a minute or two away from death.

As it turns out, my lungs had a spasm and I lost control of my breathing. It was the single, most frightening three minutes of my life. I don't remember if my life flashed before my eyes, but I do remember thinking that my time was up. But, finally it subsided and my breathing returned, albeit very labored. The attending physician now immediately admitted me of course.

I was in the hospital overnight. My family doctor came to see me in the early morning and said my breathing still sounded labored. He said he would return around lunch to determine if I would stay another day.

At around 11am, a nurse showed up with a breathing treatment. I loved those things. No one knows what asthma can be like if they haven't had it. Getting a breathing treatment is like a drug, and the wonderful ability to breathe is like a high. I always felt great after a breathing treatment. The nurse gave me the inhaler, and I happily sucked in the glorious medication until it was all gone. Ahhh...I could breathe again...

As soon as the breathing treatment was completed, the nurse gathered her equipment and left the room. Promptly, about 20 seconds later, the doctor walked in. He listened to my lungs and proclaimed that it was ok for me to go home. As I stated before, I was a meek young man. But somehow this time I found my voice.

I told him "I just had a breathing treatment."

He said, "Your lungs sound fine."

I replied, "But they didn't sound fine five minutes ago. The breathing treatment is what is making them sound fine."

He said, "There is no trace of the asthma or the pneumonia from what I can hear."

I became argumentative and told him a little more sternly, "But I was not breathing well before the treatment."

He looked at me for what seemed like several minutes, thinking. Finally, he said, "I'll make a deal with you. I'll send you to get an x-ray. If the x-ray doesn't show any signs of pneumonia, then you can go home."

This time I meekly agreed.

When I returned from x-ray, I discovered that my x-rays had already been analyzed, because as I was wheeled into my hospital room, there were three IVs and a handful of pills waiting for me. My doctor explained that the pneumonia was still there and that it had gotten much worse. He told me that he was putting me on multiple antibiotics and that I would need to spend another day or two in the hospital. Six days later, they finally released me.

Personal Case 2

When I was a young man in my early twenties, I had a terrible, debilitating back problem. I would be fine for a week or two, then suddenly, I would have severe pain in my lower left back. I could not walk correctly, and I was forced to walk with a limp. It was unbearable, and my quality of life dropped immensely. I went to my doctor and I was admitted into the hospital where I spent one week on bed rest. The doctor "diagnosed" me with spondylolisthesis, which is a condition where one of the vertebrae in the spine moves forward. This movement can cause severe pain, and if it moves enough, can cause damage to the spine.

This was wonderful! Now I knew what my problem was. Of course, the bad news that my doctor made me aware of was that it is genetic and it will be with me for the rest of my life. I would just have to learn to live with it. His medical advice was to take it easy, and if I had a flare-up, then I should lie in bed immediately until the pain subsided enough for me to get around. He called this "bed rest". Basically, to remove myself from society and my family, and just lie in bed until the pain becomes bearable again. This is what I did for several years...

Eventually, I got to the point where I wanted to try anything to make the pain go away. I consulted my doctor about seeing a chiropractor. He vehemently expressed his dissatisfaction of chiropractors, and he explained that I could further damage my spine. However, I was in my twenties and forced to live like I was in my eighties. I went against his advice and went to a chiropractor anyway.

The first chiropractor I went to was everything my doctor said it would be. He was rough and seemingly didn't care or respect my condition. He did not take any x-rays and didn't ask me any questions. However, he was the cheapest around, and I guess that proves the old adage "You get what you pay for" really does apply. I was totally unhappy with how he treated me and how he did his adjustments. I saw him that one time and never again. I told my friend about my experience, and he recommended another chiropractor that he had a good experience with. I immediately made an appointment. This chiropractor was excellent. On the first visit, he took x-rays of my back and explained how he would adjust my spine, but in a very well thought out process that would take into account my condition. On the second visit, he began questioning me about my spondylolisthesis as well as other things. I had a one hour session, and his questioning was running into the thirty minute mark. I was starting to feel frustrated. I paid for an hour session and here we are, thirty minutes in, and all we are doing is talking. When was he going to do his adjustments? I was beginning to lose confidence.

Finally, after all of his questions he asked me to do something which totally took me by surprise. He asked that I carry my wallet in my front pocket instead of my rear left pocket. Now I was young, and perception means so much when you're young. I didn't want to do it because it went against the norm. All men carry their wallets in their back pocket and I would look foolish carrying it in my front pocket. Besides, everyone else carries their wallet in their back pocket and they all don't have back conditions. I unintentionally gave him a disbelieving smirk which he immediately picked up on. He explained that he believed that my wallet was causing my spine to shift when I sat down. This shift was moving my sacrum forward in an unnatural position, which was then causing pain to my lower back. He said, "Let's just do it as an experiment." If I did not feel results in a couple of months, then I could always go back to putting my wallet in my back pocket.

His argument was convincing, and since I was there to make the pain go away, what did I have to lose? I started carrying my wallet in my front pocket and seeing the chiropractor twice a week for adjustments. With this simple change of carrying my wallet in my front pocket, and regular visits to this chiropractor, the pain was gone in two months! I have not experienced back pain since, and to this day carry my wallet in my front pocket. Had I not listened to his simple and unorthodox advice, I would probably not be writing this book sitting at my computer desk, but more likely from my bed.

Personal Case 3

When I was in my mid-thirties, I began to develop knee problems. I had difficulty walking up and down stairs. An intense pain would not allow me to bend my knees when I was going up or down stairs. The pain simply would not allow me to bend my knees. I am sure that to any observer I looked like Frankenstein going up or down stairs; I had many comments from friends and family questioning this visually obvious condition. I play guitar and keyboards and was in a band at the time. The band practiced in my cellar which means that every time we had a gig, I had to carry musical equipment up and down those stairs. Carrying the heavy amplifiers and cabinets was excruciating. However, I wasn't going to let the pain stop me from functioning. I still did the things that I needed to do, but with a tremendous amount of discomfort and pain. I went to my doctor, and he said that it could be ligament damage. I went for an x-ray, but nothing showed up that was out of the ordinary. My doctor said that I could just try pain killers or go to a specialist for possible surgery.

I wasn't looking forward to surgery, so I just put up with the pain for another six months or so until one day, as fate would have it, I was involved in a car accident. I was experiencing upper back and neck pain from the car accident, so I decided to see a chiropractor again. I had to use a different chiropractor since my old chiropractor had moved his practice to another town. This chiropractor was also very good.

My first visit was x-rays, questions, and a detailed hands-on examination of my head, neck, and upper back. No adjustments. But now I knew that this is the sign of a good chiropractor, so I was not expecting any adjustments on the first visit.

During my second visit, he began feeling the calf muscles of both of my legs. I was there for my back, but he must know what he's doing, right? He would squeeze the left side of my calf, then the right side. Then upper calf, then lower calf. Two hands on one leg, then one hand on each. After what seemed to me to be a prolonged obsession with my calves, out of the blue he said "Do you experience knee pain?" With what I am sure was an obvious surprised look, I looked at him very suspiciously. I started thinking of those people who tell you your future. You know, the ones who ask a bunch of leading questions and observe your response to tailor their next questions. This ultimately leads them to say something that seems supernatural and makes them appear like they have psychic abilities.

Now I began to feel that I am in the middle of a hoax or a scam. I quickly went over our conversations in my mind to determine what it was that I had given him, or at least clued him in on this fact. I came up with nothing. I told him that I in fact did experience knee pain. He explained that he could tell because of the difference in tension of my calf muscles. Really! My doctor never even touched my calves. This guy is telling me he can diagnose pain just by feeling the tension of my muscles. Well I did not buy that one. I again gave him a suspicious glance which he was probably looking for and quickly picked up on. He further explained that there are two muscle areas in my calf that should be relatively equal in tension if I was walking properly. But if I was not walking properly, meaning that I changed how I walk to compensate for pain, then these two muscles would have different tensions that could be discerned by a skilled observer. Finally, he said, "If you wear these orthotics that I sell, then your knee pain will go away."

There it was! The sure way into my wallet. Pick a common pain like knee pain and then claim that an insert that I put into my shoe could make it all go away. Well I wasn't parting that easily with my money. He said the orthotics shoe inserts were $300! I told him no way. I would not spend $300 on a chance... He looked at me, and he appealed to my engineering background. He told me I should be logical about it. Why put up with pain for the rest of your life when such a simple thing can make it go away? You would think that my experience with the wallet would have left me more open minded, but I still wouldn't budge. I was here for my back and neck problems, not my knee problems.

Fortunately for me, this chiropractor truly cared about his patients. Many other professionals would just chalk it up to a hard headed patient, forget about the knee issues and just move on to get paid. He looked at me for a minute, churning something over in his mind, and then he totally took me by surprise. He said, "I'll buy them. You try them for a month. If they work, you can pay me back. If not, I'll take them back and we'll call it even." How could I turn that down? This man, because he actually cares, took the money out of the equation. I told him I would be a fool not to accept his offer.

At the end of the session, he fitted me for custom orthotics. I stood on a pad with special material that collapsed under my weight. It formed a depression that was a mold of the bottom of my foot. He sent this to an orthotics manufacturer who analyzed the impression and determined where I needed support for my feet. The custom orthotics were delivered and I started wearing them. Within two weeks, my knee pain went away. Not "subsided". Not "got a little better", but totally went away. I was again dumbfounded at the simplicity of finding a root cause over masking the problem with drugs. I bought them, of course, and I have been wearing them ever since. My knee pain has never returned.

This type of issue, unfortunately, is common. I can't even imagine how many people probably have the same issue that I had. But the solution is pain killers. Mask the pain and make it bearable. Of course the pain never really totally goes away. You wind up changing the way you walk and your joints work in a way that they are not supposed to. This causes more pain, so you keep taking more pain medication. You keep making minor adjustments to how you walk and strain the joints even more, ultimately causing irreparable damage to your knees or something else. Then the final solution really is surgery.

Personal Case 4

When I was a young man, like most young men in America, I made most of my own auto repairs. And, like most home mechanics, I never had the right tools. Consequently, a repair that would take a shop four hours would take me a weekend. But I was young, and when you're young, time means nothing. So I happily wasted weekends on car repairs to save a few bucks.

On one particular occasion, I needed to change my shock absorbers. I knew I needed a special tool to remove them, but I wasn't going to spend forty or fifty dollars for a one time job. I knew I could rent the tool, but spend ten dollars for a tool that I wouldn't then own... preposterous! So, I did what every upstanding (and stupid) American young man would do, I reached for my vice grips.

Vice grips are the do all tools for home mechanics. Who needs special tools with special heads and special shapes when you have a pair of vice grips? If you're lucky, you will get the screw or offending fastener off. If not, then you will destroy the head of whatever it is you are removing. Then, in shame, you would bring it to a shop for removal. The mechanic would take one look at it and ask "Did you try to take this off yourself?" To which you would vehemently shake your head and say it must have been the previous owner. To which the mechanic would look knowingly at the shiny damaged head, with all of the freshly removed material, and promptly inform you that it was going to cost about fifty percent more than if you brought it to him in the first place. I have done this myself more than once.

This time, I was determined not to be that guy. I removed and replaced the first shock with little trouble. There was only minimal damage to the screw head and it came out fairly smoothly. It looked like it was going to be an early morning and I would be out on the lawn, basking in the sunshine for lunch.

The second shock was not as forgiving. I quickly stripped the head and it just did not want to come out. I went through various sizes of vice grips in my vice grip kit, to no avail. I tried the large one, more stripping. The small vice grip with similar results. But I was not going to allow this to get the better of me. I continued.... For hours. I know, you are thinking, "What are you? Stupid?"... Yes... Yes, I was very stupid.

I stayed in a squatting position while I furiously tried removing the shock. Now what I did not know, or ever realized, was that being in this position was actually cutting off the blood flow to my legs. When I finally was done with the shock, I stood up and felt that pins and needles, tingling sensation that you feel when you sit the wrong way and momentarily cut off the blood flow to your leg. I walked very deliberately and carefully because in those instances, the leg muscles are not quite right, and it felt like my legs would snap backwards. However, I had that feeling many times before; I wasn't worried. I finished out my day and went to bed, pleased with my success of changing the shocks.

The next morning, I got out of bed and immediately realized that the pins and needles feeling was still there. The trepidation I felt while walking was still there because my muscles still did not feel quite right. Also, I noticed that I kept tripping. A lot! I was planning on heading to the beach that day, but I was starting to get worried at this point. Especially about the tripping. I nearly fell several times and I just couldn't seem to prevent myself from tripping. It was a Sunday, so my regular doctor wasn't available; I decided to go to the emergency room.

When I saw the attending physician, he listened to my account of the previous day and immediately asked me to stand up. I stood with both feet flat on the floor. He then asked me to leave both feet flat, but then rock my left foot up with the ball of my foot remaining on the floor so that my toes pointed towards the ceiling. I did, but with great effort. And I could not get my toes very high off the floor.

Then he asked for me to do the same thing with my right foot. I looked at my foot, lying flat on the floor. My brain was commanding my toes to point up, but nothing happened. It was a very strange feeling. That is, my mind telling my foot to do something, and then my foot not doing anything. I was horrified. The doctor explained that the squatting position that I was in the previous day had cut the blood flow to my nerves and had actually damaged them to the point that they were not responding. In other words, I was partially paralyzed at my right ankle. He informed me that this was the cause of the tripping. In order to walk without tripping, you need to point your toes up every time you move your leg forward to prevent your foot from contacting the ground. My foot wouldn't point, so as I moved my right leg forward, my foot was dangling and not clearing the floor. Thus causing me to trip a lot. He called this condition "Foot Drop".

Of course, my first question was, "How long will I have this condition?" He said that the nerve is dead and I will have it for the rest of my life. I couldn't believe it. Such a stupid thing would cause lifelong damage. However, I accepted it and wound up going to the beach.

While at the beach, I was doing my best to over-exaggerate my movement on my right leg to lift it every time I moved it forward. I was doing a fairly good job. Then, while crossing the street with my young daughter, a car came towards us unexpectedly, and while trying to move quickly, I tripped. I pushed my daughter across the street, and I fell directly in the path of the car. His brakes squealed and when he finally came to a stop, he was so close that I could easily see even the smallest bug on his grill. I realized that this condition warrants a little more care and that my abilities are not what they were.

I made an appointment with my regular doctor as a follow up. I explained everything to him including what the emergency room physician said. He immediately broke out into a hearty laugh. I waited for his laughing to subside and finally he told me that my nerve, from my knee to my ankle, was in fact dead. However, the nerve is constantly growing and replacing itself. He said it would take about six months for the nerve to grow from the knee to the ankle and that I will most likely recover with no issues. I am very happy to report that he was exactly right. In just about six months, full functionality came back to both of my legs, and I have recovered fully.

My pride however, was damaged for life ☺

One More Thing

I am not writing a book about the wonders of chiropractors or about the misdeeds of doctors. Although I have some very positive experiences with chiropractors, and a few very bad experiences with doctors, my main point is that sometimes the doctors get it wrong. My experience is that ninety-nine percent of the time, the doctors get it right. It's that pesky one percent that can make all the difference in your quality of life. The old adage of "get a second opinion" is absolutely good advice. I didn't realize it then, but I know now; Get a second opinion and get it from a specialist directly related to the problem.

Getting bad news or no results from a general practitioner, and then getting the opinion of a second general practitioner may not be a good step. Seeing a specialist is well worth the peace of mind, even if you must pay extra. More importantly, the potential outcome can be much better to your health and your quality of life. This type of misdiagnosis also happened to me with my gluten symptoms. And no, a chiropractor did not figure that one out. It is even more bizarre. But I'll get to that in Chapter 3.

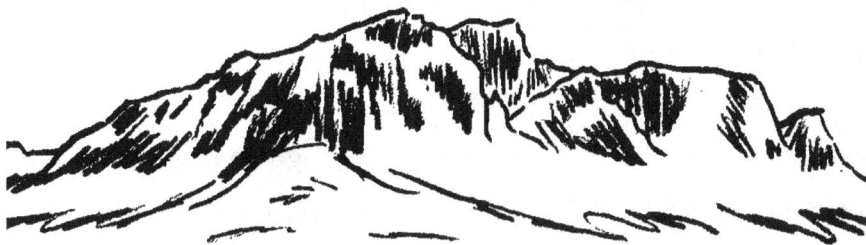

Chapter 3
Becoming Aware

My Days of Ignorance

Before I realized that I was gluten intolerant, my main symptoms were headache, nausea, and vomiting. Occasionally, these symptoms would suddenly appear and I would be nearly incapacitated. The only thing that would help is sleep; my body craved sleep during these events. If it happened while I was at work, I would have to go to my car to sleep for an hour just so I could function for the rest of the day. I was fortunate over my life that I actually had jobs that would accommodate this. I could easily see another life where I would have been losing jobs because of these symptoms and requirements.

These were not my only symptoms: I was in a fog most of the time, I constantly felt run down and lethargic, I was constipated almost all of the time, and I had a skin rash that just wouldn't go away. During the headache events, I would get bouts of acid reflux. When I tried sleeping at night, I would close my eyes, and I could see flashes of light as if it were lightning outside. When I visited the doctor during an "event", my blood pressure would be high. I lived like this for 30 years!

There were really two realizations related to my gluten intolerance. The first was figuring out what was happening to me during the headache events. The second was finally discovering that it was gluten. Let's start with how I discovered that I was experiencing migraines.

The Migraine Connection

My first memory of having a terrible headache along with the feeling of nausea is when I was about twelve years old. I was at home and I could not get out of bed. I was dizzy, nauseous, and had a terrible headache. My father worked nights, so he was home with me and my sister during the day. He was worried about me, so he brought me to our doctor who was not sure of the cause. He swabbed the back of my throat to take a culture. This immediately caused me to vomit. Miraculously, all of my symptoms went away in less than a half hour. Our family physician concluded that it was possibly a stomach bug. It sounded good at the time, but I can look back now with confidence and say, "That was definitely a migraine event".

During my twenties and thirties, I saw several different doctors about my symptoms. I went to have MRI's done. I had a CAT scan. I had an Upper GI Series. I had Ultra Sounds. I had Electro-Encephalograms. Every time I had to be examined by a new doctor, he would re-order all of the same tests. These tests on paper don't seem intrusive. But in real life, they are very intrusive. Each of these tests is typically an all-day affair. Between the preparation to go for the test, the waiting period in the office, and the test itself, I missed a day of work almost every time. For the MRI's and Electro-

Encephalograms, I was usually asked to stay awake and not sleep the night before in an attempt to cause my brain to display some kind of seizure activity. The tests showed no such activity.

During this time I discovered the power of association. One time I got sick after eating Chinese food. I associated it to the MSG, and I stopped eating Chinese food for months. Finally, I realized one day that I was still getting sick. Another time, I quickly became sick after having a bowl of cereal. I associated it to the milk. I stopped ingesting dairy for six months before I again realized that it really wasn't helping. Finally, my doctor said it was probably whey. I stopped eating anything that had whey for six months with no change in my symptoms.

You might ask, "Why would you do that for so long?" But the fact is, when you feel as poorly as I did, you want to believe. You really want to believe that you found the problem, and now your life is going to change for the better. When I was eliminating dairy and I got sick, I would immediately try to think of what dairy I must have accidentally ingested. When I stopped eating whey and I became sick, I read the ingredients of everything I was eating. I wanted desperately to believe that one of these food items was causing my health problems. Ultimately though, my hopes would always be dashed, and my illness always returned.

In my forties, I saw a doctor who gave it a try by ordering all of the usual tests. He found nothing, but he did find my case interesting. He presented it to the hospital round table - A group of doctors that looked at and discussed the more difficult cases. They decided to send me to a neurologist for the "events" and to an ear, nose, and throat doctor for my acid reflux and dizziness.

I saw the Ear, Nose, and Throat doctor only once, and he promptly diagnosed me with IBS. I had never heard of IBS, so he gave me a pamphlet on it. It stands for Irritable Bowel Syndrome. What I realize now is that IBS is a catch-all for something that cannot be explained related to digestion. Sorry doc, IBS sounded great to someone who was desperately looking for an answer, but I am fairly certain that you got that one wrong.

I saw the neurologist. He was the first to call them "episodes" because he did not have a diagnosis for it. He put me through the usual battery of tests. After a few visits, he determined that I was experiencing seizures. He did not have any proof from the tests, but my episodes were classic symptoms of seizures. Seizures... scary, but at least now I knew what my problem was. He decided to put me on anti-seizure medication called Topomax[ii]. I took the Topomax per his instructions. The following evening I was at band practice learning a new song on my guitar. The other guitarist was showing me a lick and my mind could not translate it to my hands. I felt totally confused, and I couldn't get my mind to make my hands work. It was like my foot drop all over again. Except the paralysis was being caused by medecine. I left practice early and did not take any more Topomax.

The next day, I called the neurologist and told him about my Topomax experience. He said that, yeah, sometimes that happens. He said maybe I should stop taking the Topomax. I told him that I was way ahead of him, and I had no plans on taking any more. He said that it is best to stop gradually (the initial doses were four pills). There was no way I was going to maintain that kind of confusion, so I just stopped.

They Are Called Migraines...

While I was waiting for my next appointment at the neurologist, I decided to do some investigation on my own. I entered all of my symptoms into Google, and what came back was "migraine". What I discovered, not from any doctor, but through the power of the internet is that I was experiencing migraines.

During that month, thanks to the Mayo Clinic website[iii], I learned more about migraines than I ever wanted to. Most people think of migraines as just headaches, but in reality there are four stages to a migraine. People can experience one, some, or all of the stages.

The first stage is called the Prodrome. This is the stage where a person would feel the migraine coming on. That person would get very lethargic and also begin to feel nauseous. This would happen to me, and this stage would last anywhere from two to forty-eight hours.

The second stage is the Aura. Aura is basically a hallucination. It is a neurological reaction to the migraines effect on the brain. 95% of people that experience Aura experience it as an optical hallucination. They see flashes of light, even with their eyes open. I experienced this, but only with my eyes closed. My main Aura came in the form of an olfactory hallucination. I would get a "smell" in my nose that would be there no matter where I was. It smelled to me like burning metal. When this happened to me, the fear of a migraine was always at the front of my mind. At least 80% of the time that I experienced Aura, it would turn into a migraine headache. Certain odors, always manmade odors, to this day will trigger an aura. That aura will now, on rare occasions, still turn into a migraine. It makes me wonder if all of those years of eating gluten and getting migraines didn't somehow train my brain to react adversely to these odors.

The third stage is the actual migraine headache attack. It is a terrible thing to experience. Many people believe that they have migraines, but migraines are debilitating. A migraine headache can make a person lose their capacity to think. To lose their ability to socialize. Light is uncomfortable... Bright lights are downright painful. Sunlight is torture. Loud sounds make your head feel like someone just hit you with a hammer. A dark room with no sound is usually the preference of a migraine sufferer during a migraine headache.

I was in the hospital once for a cut that needed stitching. As I sat there, a young girl came in and I overheard her tell the receptionist that she had a migraine headache and needed a shot to make it go away. I was full into my gluten free diet by then and I wasn't even aware that there was a shot for migraine sufferers. I watched as the young girl of about 18 sat totally engrossed in a book that she brought with her. She appeared well prepared for the wait. I got the feeling that she had done this at least a few times before. She sat very comfortably, and she never showed any signs of distress. Eventually she got up, and she went to the vending machine and got some potato chips. She enjoyed the potato chips while she read some more. I am sure that she probably had a headache, and in her mind she really believed that she had a migraine. But take it from me... I seriously doubt that she had a migraine headache. A migraine is the worst part of my symptoms. Everything else is uncomfortable, but a migraine headache makes me want to leave the human race for a while and sit in total seclusion. Watching that girl in the emergency room, draining valuable resources for what certainly appeared not to be an emergency, makes me wonder about our healthcare system. But that's another book☺

The fourth stage is the Post-drome. This stage on the one hand, is pleasurable to get to because it means the migraine headache is now gone. On the other hand, it brings its own terrible symptoms. Mainly lethargy and the urge to sleep. Long sleep. For me, thirteen to twenty hours straight. When I would finally feel like actually getting out of bed, I would feel great. I would generally be hungry, and all of the fog would be lifted. But the hours in bed were in a total, unthinking fog. No dreams, no thinking, just sleep as if I were put under for a tooth extraction. I look back at all of the wasted hours. But then

I look forward with bliss knowing that those terrible, horrible days are now far behind me.

When I went back to the neurologist, I told him what I discovered about my symptoms and migraines. Part way into my appointment, I told him that I had an episode the previous week. He told me, "Let's not call it that anymore. Let's call it what it is... a migraine." This is someone who was probably making thirty times my pay for his expertise, and how do I discover the name of my malady? Google, of course! He decided at that point to send me to a Migraine Clinic. This is a specialized clinic that treats migraine sufferers only. Thus only people that suffered with migraines went there. So, after self-diagnosing my migraines, I went to the clinic.

The doctor was nice enough. He had me keep a diary of things I ate so that we could determine if food was the problem. During my time here, I was never able to find a connection to my migraines and what I ate. He, like his predecessors, determined that it must be seizures. He ordered an MRI. It came back negative, but it *MUST* be seizures. He put me on an anti-seizure drug called Depakote[iv]. I promptly gained 40 pounds and my migraines were worse than ever.

At this point, my migraines were happening about three times a week now. The doctor also put me on another migraine medication called Zomig[v]. When I felt a migraine coming on, I was to take one Zomig. I did as directed. After ingesting the Zomig, I would feel a strange burning sensation at the base of my neck. I would feel like I just got hit by a truck, but sometimes the migraine would go away. This is yet another odd thing about western medicine. You get drugs to treat an original symptom, but this drug causes side effects, so the doctor gives you drugs to treat the side effects, which in turn cause different side effects, so the doctor prescribes yet another drug, and so on and on and on... Next thing you know, you are like my father-in-law, taking a fistful of pills twice a day. The Zomig offered an interesting dilemma... Keep the migraine or get hit by a truck. I chose the truck, but a couple of months into it, the Zomig didn't help anymore. So for a while I just felt like someone with a migraine that got hit by a truck.

I have never said this to a soul, but at that point in my life, suicide actually began creeping into my thoughts. I never would do that because of my family. I could never put them through that, but just the idea of living like this for another 30 or 40 years made me as sick as the migraines themselves. I was extremely depressed. Unfortunately, my friends and family were not much help. I don't blame them; they didn't understand. No one can know what a person goes through with a migraine without actually experiencing it. My family and friends would offer their solutions: "It is stress... you need to learn to relax!", "It's mold in your house. That happened to a friend I know.", "You are eating too much red meat", "You shouldn't be eating any meat", "You should work out more", You don't get enough sleep." I have heard them all. Everyone has an opinion on the cause.

Then one day, I figured out a way to "control" the migraines. Don't eat when I started feeling poorly. If it got worse, then allow myself to vomit. As disgusting as that is, it would help me feel better. I could at least function. During these migraines, I was extremely nauseous. What I didn't know then, but what I realize now, is that is my body was trying to purge the gluten. In the beginning I would fight the urge. After all, who wants to vomit! But what I understand now, is that by fighting this urge, the gluten remained in my system and was forced to exit through my digestive tract. What that translates to is my symptoms being amplified and the symptoms lasting for days instead of hours. I lived like this for another two years. And then it happened….

I Am Gluten Intolerant

September 2012, a month I will never forget. It was coincidence, or as I like to believe, serendipity. I was at the gym trying to lose my newly acquired 40 pounds. I was on the treadmill jogging. In this gym, like in most gyms, they have televisions to watch while on the treadmill. However, you are a captive audience. You have to watch the station that is on. That particular day, Doctor Oz was on[vi]. As I started jogging I thought, "Oh great! Just my luck!" To me these afternoon shows are like watching a soap opera; not my cup of tea. I looked at the other televisions, and a few had the news on. I contemplated moving to one with the news, but luckily, I was feeling particularly lazy that day (at the gym, no less☺), and I decided to just watch the Doctor Oz show. It was the single best and most important decision I have ever made in my life.

What I discovered during that show was that I had many of the symptoms of gluten intolerance. Including migraines, nausea, vomiting, IBS, skin rash, brain fog, and feeling lethargic. As I listened to their description of the symptoms, I thought, "That's me!" As soon as I got home I began to research gluten. Similar to my experience with migraines, I found that there was a vast amount of material related to gluten. All of it pointing to me possibly having gluten sensitivity.

One thing I could not find was any reference to a test that would prove gluten sensitivity. I was unwilling, because of all of my previous experiences, to go to my doctor just to start another ridiculous round of tests. I decided at that point to eliminate gluten from my diet as an experiment. What I did not realize, is just how difficult that would be, and how difficult that is even to this day.

An interesting side note... Once I discovered that eating gluten free was making my symptoms disappear, I told my doctor that I believed all of my years of suffering were due to gluten. He told me he was happy to hear that. I asked him what I should do and what should I stay away from. He told me, "There is a wealth of information online for gluten free diets. If you do some research, you will find a diet that you can follow".

Really? I had to diagnose myself, and now I have to research online to determine a diet for myself? Even just a little guidance would have been appreciated. Of course the doctor bill for that visit was right on time in my mailbox ☺

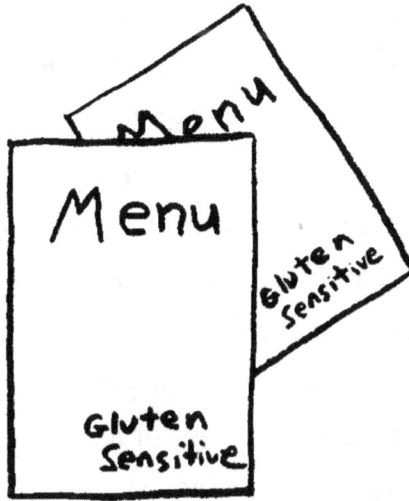

Chapter 4
Becoming Gluten Free at Restaurants

Going It Alone

When I first started my journey to become gluten free, it was not as prevalent and in the forefront as it is today. There were very few restaurants that offered gluten free items and the supermarkets had close to nothing. It is during my first 8 months that I made my first big mistake. That is, not discussing with the chef or server about my gluten intolerance. I tried to do it on my own.

I tried to be intelligent about it. For instance, I knew that meat does not have gluten. Therefore, steaks, chicken, pork, etc. are all fine to ingest. One particular restaurant had very good steaks. I ate there several times, getting sick every time. I blamed it on the potatoes because maybe they put some kind of filler in them that contained wheat. I blamed it on something I ate before the meal that maybe I was unaware of. I tried to blame everything except the steak.

Of course, I couldn't see any reason why gluten would be in steak, but at a deeper level, I did not want to have to give up yet another food item that I really enjoyed eating. Eventually, I stopped going there for a while. I went back when the restaurant became more gluten aware, and I discovered that the flavoring that was put onto the steak had gluten in it as a thickening agent. I ordered a steak with salt and pepper only and had no issues.

As a side note, I also discovered that the corn also had a sauce on top that contained gluten. So two items that I would have figured were safe both had gluten. I never would have figured it out at the time, because I always ordered the corn or the steak. You can see how easily you can be tricked if you try to go it alone.

Gluten *Sensitive* Menus

Another local restaurant prides themselves in catering to people with food allergies. I ate there a couple of times. The food was great, and I had no problems. Occasionally, they would change the menu to mix it up and offer new items.

On one particular day, they offered a nice shrimp scampi with gluten free noodles. I knew the gluten free noodles were nowhere near as good as the wheat, but sometimes a restaurant can pull it off pretty well. I was there with my wife at the time, who was not gluten free, and she ordered the shrimp scampi, but with wheat noodles. This place does a fine job for gluten intolerant patrons. The manager delivers the order in a special square plate to indicate that it is gluten free.

I tried mine and couldn't believe how good it tasted and how they had managed to get the noodles to have what appeared to be nearly the consistency of wheat. Well, as you probably guessed, that evening - and the following day - I had a violent migraine with all of the symptoms. The migraine was unbelievably intense. I couldn't get out of bed for two days. When the fog lifted and I was back to my senses, I realized that somehow the restaurant must have delivered the wrong meal. I told my wife of my suspicion, and she then told me how bad she thought her noodles were. It became clear that somehow the restaurant, even with their internal safe guards, still managed to mix up our orders. We are all human, and sometimes mistakes happen. I did not hold it against the restaurant, but the next time I went in I did let the manager know about my experience. The manager was extremely pleasant and promised to be more careful. I have had to inform managers several times, and they are not all as pleasant...

On another occasion, I had dinner at a popular restaurant chain. They actually listed the gluten free items on the menu, but in a different color. The idea is that the restaurant can make it gluten free, but regular menu items may not be gluten free. This can be the most dangerous type, because you are putting your faith in the server that they will get it right when reporting it to the cook. On this occasion, I got what I thought was a pretty safe steak meal. Unfortunately, I became very ill with my classic gluten symptoms. The following week I went back to the restaurant and informed the manager of what transpired the previous week. I was extremely courteous as I always am about such things. Here is basically how the conversation went.

Me: I just wanted to let you know that I had dinner here last week. I am gluten intolerant, and I ordered a gluten free meal. I became sick and I believe that the cook or server might have accidentally made an error with my meal. I just want to make you aware that an accidental mistake might have occurred.

Manager: I am not giving you a free meal!

Me: (With an obvious look of surprise on my face) I was not asking for a free meal. I just wanted to let you know, because some people like myself can actually become sick from gluten.

Manager: We don't make those kind of mistakes. We are careful, and I am not giving you anything for free.

Me: (Now quite upset) I know from past experience that accidents can happen. You understand that I came here to give this restaurant a second chance and never once mentioned anything about a free meal. I am leaving now and I will never return.

Manager: You do what you have to do.

Most restaurants, in fact nearly all restaurants, franchise or privately owned, do not treat customers like this. But occasionally, you get a bad manager. I held true to my promise and I have never stepped foot into that restaurant again. Frankly, even if he became pleasant at the end of the conversation, I would never believe that he would take the gluten free requirements seriously.

Maybe It Wasn't the Restaurant Food...

One question I frequently get when I recount my experiences is, "How do you know it was the restaurant food? Maybe it was something else."

What people don't realize is that I have a lifetime of experience that lets me know exactly what is happening with my body. I know all of the symptoms and the signs now. When I eat something and my stomach starts to become queasy within a half an hour, then I have ingested some hardcore gluten and I better purge it as quickly as possible. If I fight it, then a full blown migraine along with heavy sleep, lethargy, constipation, nausea, and severe headache will be the outcome. If I ingest small amounts of gluten, it can actually be worse for me. When this happens, I don't get the quick upset stomach. Instead I will unwittingly go to bed and wake up to the alarm still feeling very sleepy with the beginnings of a migraine headache in the back of my head.

I try to purge at this point, but it is too late. The food that I ate is past my stomach and is now in my digestive tract. Now I have to wait for it to go through my system on its own. That means a day or two of feeling very ill, sleepy, constipated, and with a migraine headache. The migraine is not as severe as if I ate a lot of gluten, but it is a migraine nonetheless, and it is very uncomfortable. For me, at this point in my life, eating a little gluten is far worse than eating a lot.

While I am on this point, there is something to be said about thresholds. Before I was aware that I had gluten intolerance, I ate gluten. I ate a lot of gluten. I ate bread, pasta, pastries, and more. What I have come to realize is that at that time, I had a much higher tolerance for gluten. I could eat things without getting sick. However, when I did get sick, it was very bad. I never could quite pinpoint the actual foods that caused my illness. Sometimes I would eat a pastry without getting sick, and other times I would eat the same pastry and get sick. So in my mind, it couldn't be the pastry, or it would have always made me sick.

I know now that my threshold was constantly moving up and down depending on how much gluten was in my system. So on some occasions, I would eat something and it would not be enough to push me over my threshold to actually become sick. Other times I would eat the very same thing, but it would be enough to push me over my threshold, and I would become sick. Because of this, my quest to find a root cause was always a moving target. Looking back, it's no wonder that I could not pinpoint it to any one food item. Today, my threshold is very low. If I have one small piece of bread it can trigger a severe migraine.

Once, I went to a restaurant in Connecticut while staying in a hotel at Foxwoods Casino, and I discovered just how low my tolerance threshold now is. The restaurant offered some gluten free turkey soup. For anyone who is attempting to be gluten free, you would understand that soup is a food item that is almost never listed on a gluten free menu. The noodles are obviously one issue, but another problem is that the soup is very often thickened by putting some wheat flour into the broth. So when I heard that I could have gluten free soup, I jumped at the chance.

I have to admit that the soup was quite delicious. I was finished gambling for the night, and it was fairly late in the evening. I was tired, and I wanted a quick meal before bed. I hungrily downed the soup, and I went to the hotel room to go to sleep.

When I tried to get up in the morning, I could not get out of bed. My head was absolutely pounding with the worst, most painful migraine headache that I have ever experienced. I wanted to sleep... desperately I needed sleep, but the excruciating headache kept preventing me from going into a deep sleep. The racking and throbbing kept me from falling asleep, and I kept squeezing different parts of my head with my hands to attempt to stop the pain. It was my last night at the hotel, and I had to be out by 2pm. At about 1pm, I forced myself out of bed, and took a quick shower. I was still feeling like I got hit by a train, but I forced myself out of the hotel.

Gradually, I started feeling a little better. I decided that I would go to the restaurant to determine if something could have happened that was gluten related. When I got to the restaurant, I asked the manger about the turkey soup. He said he was sure that it was gluten free. The soup is all that I had the previous evening. I was sure there was something in the soup. I persisted, and I asked what the ingredients were in the soup. He listed turkey, peas, carrots, onions, celery, broth, salt, pepper... and then he said something that took me by surprise, but at the same time, I was not surprised. He said that they cook the soup with wheat noodles, but they remove them to make the soup gluten free. Bingo! And that was my first experience with cross contamination.

Cross Contamination

Cross contamination is when a food that has gluten contaminates a food that does not have gluten. That was my first experience. I have had several other experiences as well. I have been sickened by french fries. Most restaurants, I now know, unfortunately cook things like chicken nuggets with wheat breading along with gluten free french fries. Once the fries are cooked, they are also now covered in gluten.

On another occasion, I went to an outdoor ice cream shop. I asked about the ice cream and about the chocolate hot fudge. They had documentation listing what is gluten free. That is always a nice bonus at a restaurant or an ice cream shop when you are gluten intolerant. I selected a gluten free flavor with the gluten free hot fudge. It was very good, because it is locally made ice cream. However, after eating it, I promptly became sick. The next time I went to the ice cream shop, I was naturally apprehensive about ordering ice cream again. Finally, however, I decided I would go with the safe vanilla flavor and no topping.

While I was standing in line, I was watching the workers as they swiftly made and delivered the ice cream to dozens of people. These workers are mainly high-school and college kids. They work very hard and extremely fast. While watching one of these workers make a hot fudge sundae, the hot fudge pot caught my eye. I watched in horror as workers were grabbing ladles full of hot fudge, and thrusting them into any, and all kinds of ice cream. The ladles, still dripping with ice cream like Cookies and Cream, a gluten bomb, were inserted back into the hot fudge. Of course I got sick! The gluten free hot fudge was not gluten free at all. The workers had inadvertently turned the gluten free hot fudge into a cross contaminated gluten nightmare. I don't blame the workers, they just don't understand cross contamination or the consequences of people who are gluten intolerant.

This was a big lesson for me. Cross contamination is something that anyone who is gluten intolerant has to really pay attention to. Many servers do not understand the concept and more importantly, do not understand the consequences. Always ask the right questions, and if you don't like the answers or if the server doesn't appear knowledgeable about gluten, then that is a sign that you might want to go with the salad.

Speaking of salads, we all know that vegetables are gluten free. However, many, many salad dressings are not. In fact, in my experiences with restaurants, very few salad dressings are gluten free. I have become sick more than once by eating salad dressing at a restaurant. Also, most restaurants offer croutons on their salads. You must be certain that they are not just taking a pre-made salad, removing the croutons, and then serving it to you. This is yet another form of cross contamination that can be disastrous.

Food Servers

My general rule is, if the server is unsure about what the restaurant offers that is gluten free, or they use words like "I think that's gluten free", or "I'm pretty sure that doesn't have gluten", then your safe play is to order a salad. However, if you couldn't trust the server about the gluten content of a meal, then why trust them about the gluten content of a salad dressing? So, in these situations I order a plain salad, no croutons, and no salad dressing. I also make sure that the server informs the chef that I have a gluten allergy.

Informing the server does not necessarily mean that all is now well. If the server is thoughtful and well intentioned, then you have nothing to worry about. Fortunately, that describes 95% of all servers. But there are servers that are misguided or that simply could not care less. Those are:

The Clueless Ones

They have not heard of gluten. They don't care about gluten. As you speak, their eyes are darting around and there is usually a smile on their face that reminds you of the smile you give grandma when you tell her you like the pajamas she bought you for Christmas. As you tell them to let the chef know about your gluten allergy, they nod their head yes, but don't write anything down. They, like, also, you know, like, say like, like a lot. If you get one of these servers, be wary. Look over your meal before ingesting or you could be in for a long day tomorrow.

The know-it-all

This is the server who already knows everything you have to say. They constantly interrupt you so they can finish what you are saying.

Me: Yes, I would like the salad, but...

Server: Don't worry, I won't have them put on croutons

Me: Actually, I was going to ask about...

Server: We won't put bread crumbs or anything with bread in it

Me: Yes, that's good. What I wanted to ask is do you have gluten free salad dressing

Server: Oh... I'm pretty sure everything we have is gluten free

Me: Can you ask the chef please?

Yeah, the "pretty sure" thing is a clue that the salad dressing might not be a safe bet. Of course, I would request that they ask the chef, and then you can judge the quality of the response. My experience is that the vast majority of the time, the chef is knowledgeable with gluten related questions.

Generally, these servers are actually knowledgeable, however, they tend to be sloppy. They lull you into a false sense of security, and you let your guard down. They ultimately forget something in the chain of custody for your order, and you will pay with a day in bed.

The "Overly Friendly" Server

Think of the server with way more than 25 pieces of Flair in the movie Office Space. These are the servers that sit right next to you on your very first visit. Or kneel down so they are eye to eye with you. They are loud, overly friendly, and this can be quite uncomfortable. These servers are just trying (very hard) to make your experience more pleasurable by attempting to insert themselves at a more personal level. They don't mean any disservice and for the most part, once you get past the invasion of your personal space, they can be quite entertaining and pleasant.

My only problem with this type of server is that with the boisterous and fast-paced personality, they tend to want to move very quickly. They want to get your drinks fast, they want to get the food fast, and herein lies the problem. They want to take your order fast. So fast that sometimes I feel that they are not hearing my concerns about gluten. In the beginning days of my gluten free restaurant experience, I would let these servers control the pace. After several gluten mishaps, I now know to take control of the pace. Slow them down a bit to make sure, through several repeated questions, that my concerns are heard, and more importantly, understood.

The "I Obviously Hate My Job" server

These are the servers who have a look on their face like they just smelled a skunk. If you ask any questions, gluten related or otherwise, they sigh and give you the impression that you are keeping them from something very important and this "order" is just getting in their way. If you ask what they have for sides, unlike most servers who bother to take the time and memorize them, these servers will flip through your menu in front of your face and point like a caveman to the page with the sides. If you ask if the steak has anything gluten in it, they would say "Yeah, I think so". It's an easy answer so they don't have to walk all the way to the chef to find out for sure. Do not trust these servers. Even if they went to ask the chef a question for me, I can't bring myself to trust the answer.

Just to be clear, 95% of all servers are great. They are trustworthy, very nice, like theirs jobs, and really are trying to make your dining experience pleasurable. Occasionally, I'll get that outstanding one who is extremely knowledgeable, remembers you, has a great personality, and cares about getting your gluten free order correct. When this happens, I get their name and I request them every time I return to that restaurant. If you are gluten free or not, I believe this is always a good practice anyway. Dining out at a restaurant becomes much more pleasurable when you can develop a pleasurable relationship with your server. Many of them will bring our favorite drinks to our table without even asking. They know what we usually order. They remember our names. We know a little about them, and they know a little about us. It makes for an excellent environment. My advice would be to always get to know your servers, requesting them whenever you can.

By the way, I know that gluten intolerance is not technically considered an allergy, but why try to explain this nuance to the servers? Everyone understands allergy... So I always just say that I have a gluten allergy. Keep it simple and straight forward, and there is less chance of your server getting it wrong.

Unexplained Events

Finally, let me discuss the worst part for me about eating out at a restaurant. I'll start with a few examples.

A local popular chicken franchise offers a decent gluten free roasted chicken breast along with gluten free sides. I always get the roasted chicken breast with corn and potatoes. No bread and no gravy. I ate this combination here for a couple of years and had no issues. One day, about six months ago, I ordered this plate, and the next morning I had my classic headache and lethargy. I know that all of the other things I ingested the previous day were not the cause because they came from my own home which is 100% gluten free. So, I was positive that the migraine came from the meal at the restaurant.

I made my choices based on an online menu that lists all of the items in this restaurant that are gluten free, according to the manufacturer, not the restaurant. In fact, in order to see the menu online, you have to check that you agree with an online statement that basically states that there can be cross contamination on any of the usual allergens including gluten. However, this is typical for restaurants nowadays. They want to inform us of allergens and try to make our dining experience pleasurable by keeping the allergens away, but they always make it clear that there can be cross contamination for liability reasons. In other words, they are saying that you are taking a chance and that it is risky to eat there. But they have to say that in today's litigious environment. People have sued restaurants for much less, so they have to try to cover themselves for the inevitable accident of cross contamination.

Another popular franchise offers cafeteria style options with Southwestern food. You can get a wrap, bowl, or salad, and you choose the sides. When I inform them of my gluten allergy, they tell me that there are only a couple of the sauces that are off limits. All of the vegetables, meat, and rice are gluten free.

I usually order the white rice, chicken, and various vegetables. I have eaten there several times with no issues. They, of course, always have the disclaimer that they are not a gluten free restaurant, and there is always a chance of cross contamination. But unfortunately, that is always a risk if you want to dine out when you have a food allergy.

One time I ordered the brown rice, and everything else was the same. The next morning was migraine and lethargy for the entire day. On this particular occasion, I had eaten some other things during the day that were not from my home. So, since my experience at the Southwestern Style restaurant had always been good, I determined that the issue must have been one of the other items.

I had only eaten half of the Southwestern Bowl that I had ordered from the restaurant and I put the remainder in the refrigerator. A couple of days later, I decided to eat the rest of the food for lunch. By dinner, I was sick, and I realized that it was the Southwestern Bowl causing the problem. I was fortunate that time because I realized it before going to bed. So I was able to purge it from my system, thus avoiding the headache and lethargy the following day.

This, of course, leads to the power of association again. I will still eat at the restaurant, but I do not know if it was the brown rice or if there was cross contamination. I have no interest in experimenting to find out, so I simply will not order the brown rice again.

On another occasion, I ordered a meal at a regular Southwestern Style restaurant. I ordered a chicken meal that is gluten free anyway with the exception of tortilla strips that are placed on top. I have been to this restaurant many times, and I had ordered this particular meal several times before.

On this particular occasion, I got a few bites into my meal when, to my horror, I saw a tortilla strip in my meal. That is very scary for me because I know what it could potentially mean if I would have ingested it.

I immediately notified the manager, who was very pleasant and extremely apologetic. He removed my plate, and brought another meal, as well as taking the meal off of the bill. That was a nice gesture, but my worry was getting sick.

Fortunately, I did not get sick that time. But, it highlights just how easily an accident can happen. Someone in the kitchen accidentally put that in. I firmly believe it was an accident, and I am fully aware that things like that can happen. There is always a risk when dining out. Anyone who holds the restaurant responsible, in my opinion is foolish because eventually an accident like this is bound to happen no matter what procedures are put in place. What ultimately determines whether or not I go back is the manager's reaction to a mistake. In this case, I believe the manager did a fine job, and I still go to this restaurant to this day.

These types of incidents also occur at restaurants that I have had good experiences with. I start dining there, and I'll go several times with no issues. Then suddenly, I will have a problem with one experience. I then go back and again have no issues. It is a frustrating, risky business. I am putting myself into the hands of others to keep my meals gluten free.

The problem, of course, is that the people in the chain of custody do not understand what happens when someone is exposed. If they experienced what I experience with gluten, then they would take better care when preparing meals. But to many of them, gluten intolerance, or allergies in general, are just a minor inconvenience that causes a rash or some other insignificant symptom. So they just don't have the understanding. Thus, the will is not there to give the extra effort that would ensure that a meal is free of allergens.

Again, I don't blame them. It is human nature. I don't expect them to understand what I go through. I don't expect them to care about the gluten the way that I do. If I did, I would be a fool, and I would be setting myself up for massive disappointment. My view is that it is up to me to try and understand who is serving me and how seriously the restaurant takes my allergy. If I don't get the impression that the restaurant takes gluten seriously, or that my server really has no clue and doesn't care, then it is up to me to modify what I want along with what I am willing to eat from that restaurant. Or, even if I want to stay or ever come back.

There have also been many restaurants that claim that meals are gluten free, and I get sick the very first time I eat there. In these cases, the power of association is too much for me, and I just can't bring myself to eat there again. Fortunately, or unfortunately, if I have a bad experience the very first time, I will never go back. Well, never say never... I will give it a good long time, and they will have to demonstrate to me that they have gotten their act together regarding allergies.

Dining Out Is a Risky Business

All of these examples underscore the fact that cross contamination is a very real risk, and that it does, and *WILL*, happen. My desire to dine out is fairly strong. There is something about going to a nice restaurant, enjoying the company of friends and family, and not having to worry about cooking and cleaning. It is an experience that I am not willing to give up.

So, with all of this knowledge and experience, I have to accept the fact that if I plan to dine out in the future, I will continue to sometimes have gluten related contamination, and I will continue to have all of the symptoms that go along with that. It is my choice. All I can do is to be as diligent as I possibly can, go to the restaurants that I trust the most, and make menu choices that I know make the most sense to avoid gluten.

I guess my advice to anyone with gluten intolerance, or any other allergies, is to balance the risk with your desire to dine out. My risk is a terrible, painful, and uncomfortable feeling. But it is not life threatening. If I had a peanut allergy that could potentially close my airways due to a cross contamination accident, I don't think that I could put that into the hands of teenage kitchen workers and servers at restaurants.

I have a response to gluten that is very uncomfortable. However, I also feel that I have become so tuned in to my body's reactions to gluten, that I can safely accept the risk of eating out. I now know fairly quickly if I have ingested a substantial amount of gluten that is going to cause terrible symptoms the following day. I have the option to purge this, which I will do just to keep the symptoms at bay. The reaction itself, the upset stomach and nausea, are my body's way of telling me to get to the nearest bathroom and purge this poison.

So, I am willing to accept the risk. I thoroughly enjoy dining out, and I have a short list of restaurants that I thoroughly trust. I have good experiences with the management. They are willing to listen and improve, and that keeps me coming back. I stick with trusted servers, and I have a list of meals that I enjoy and that I have had few issues with.

There is no reason why we should not go out and enjoy a nice meal at a restaurant just because you are gluten intolerant. But it takes awareness, diligence, and intelligent choices to try and keep yourself symptom free.

Gluten Free vs. Gluten Sensitive

One final observation about restaurants. When I first became aware that I was gluten intolerant, there were very few restaurants with gluten free menus. Then suddenly many restaurants offered gluten FREE menus. Then, just as suddenly, the menus changed to gluten SENSITIVE menus. I know, it is a nuance, but this minor distinction helps to relieve the restaurant from liability. Where I used to get responses like "Yes, we are gluten free", I now get, "Well, we offer a gluten sensitive menu. We do not guarantee that we are gluten free. Cross contamination can occur anywhere, even in the air with flour dust."

In reality, this is true. In today's litigious society, can you blame them? So it really doesn't bother me that they say this. My question after these types of responses is, "Do you have a procedure to minimize the gluten exposure?" If they give me a resounding "Yes" with confidence, then I am ok with it.

Going it alone in a restaurant is never the correct method to choose. I am not sure if I attempted to analyze the menu without notifying the restaurant because I was embarrassed, if I was ashamed of my condition, or if I just felt like I knew what I was doing. Either way, it is the wrong way! What I have learned is to always notify the server that you have a gluten allergy. Then, always gauge their response to determine if they are knowledgeable and trustworthy.

Just remember that most servers do not understand the ramifications of getting it wrong. Ultimately, it is up to *you* to take control when dining out at a restaurant.

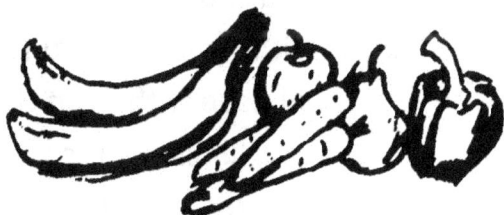

Chapter 5
Becoming Gluten Free at Home

Eating at home is now the safest and most stress free way for me to have dinner. I live alone at this point, and I am able to make everything in my house gluten free. However, it was, and still is, not always easy. When I first became gluten free, I was not living alone, and it is definitely much more problematic.

The easiest items to eat, of course, are fruits, vegetables, and meat. All fruit, all vegetables, and all meat is naturally gluten free. What makes it a challenge is understanding if there are toppings, sauces, fillers, or dressings involved.

If you get meat that is still on the bone and there is no added flavoring, then you are nearly one hundred percent sure that it is safe. If, however, there is flavoring or a topping, like barbeque sauce or teriyaki sauce, then gluten may be inside. You should look for gluten free on the package or check with the manufacturer to be sure.

Another potential issue with meat is if it has been rolled or processed. Think lunch meat or kielbasa. Sometimes the manufacturer will put a wheat based filler to either help bind the meat together, or simply just to fill it with something cheaper than meat to get the volume up. This is a sneaky way to lower the cost or a way to give it a nicer consistency. Either way, it could spell disaster if you are not careful. You definitely want to be sure you get confirmation that the ingredients are in fact gluten free or the next morning you will probably not be getting out of bed.

As long as there is no salad dressing, then vegetables are one hundred percent ok. Vegetables and fruits are naturally gluten free, and the only way for them to have gluten is through contact from the outside. Of course, they should be washed, but I would do that with any fresh vegetable or fruit anyway, regardless of allergies.

The Ingredient List Helps... Sometimes

Dressings can be a challenge. Actually, anything in a bottle or can may be challenging. If the manufacturer doesn't list gluten free on the bottle or can, then it could be a game of Russian Roulette. Manufacturers are becoming more aware of gluten, but some still don't list allergy ingredients. Also, some things, like vinegar and soy sauce, can actually contain gluten. So, if the ingredients don't list wheat, rye, barley, or triticale specifically, there are other ingredients that could actually contain gluten. With these types of labels, you should always find it on the manufacturer's website or send the manufacturer a letter to request the information. If you don't want to be bothered with finding this out, then it is a crap shoot. You can eat the dressing or whatever it may be, and hope for the best. If symptoms don't appear, then you can add another food to your gluten free list. If symptoms do appear, then it will suck being you for about three days.

I have tried the crap shoot method, and I have added some foods, and much to my dismay, I have eliminated some foods. Of course, to eliminate the foods, I paid dearly with a migraine, nausea, and digestive issues. As I become more experienced, I am far less likely to attempt the crap shoot method. Although occasionally, my senses leave me, and I talk myself into believing that something that I really want must be gluten free. Of course, it turns out not to be gluten free, and I pay again with a three day mind fog.

And…. Embarrassingly, I sometimes just don't learn. I love pistachios. I found a company that has gluten free listed on the package, so I was in my glory. I happily consumed a quarter of the bag and the next morning my head was ready to explode from the pain.

I suspected the pistachios, but, hey, it said gluten free! So, about a week later, I tried some more; I was rewarded with yet another painful headache. I stopped eating them, and I threw them away. I learned my lesson, right? Wrong! A few months later, I explained to myself that it couldn't be the pistachios. After all, the bag says "gluten free!" So I made a third attempt, which, of course, delivered my third migraine. Three strikes, and you're out for sure. That was a while ago, and so far, I have not lost my senses enough to go for a fourth round.

This highlights two things. The first being my stupidity. I know that they are causing it, but my desire to have that delightful pistachio overwhelms my senses, making me stupid. There is no other excuse. It reminds me just how difficult it can be to give up some of my favorite foods by going gluten free.

Manufacturer Gluten Free Labeling

The second thing is labeling. According to the United States Food and Drug Administration website, the government requirement to be able to label something as either "gluten free", "free of gluten", "no gluten", or "without gluten", is that the maximum amount of gluten that a food can contain is less than 20 ppm (parts per million)[vii]. This is a very small amount. The reason for this particular amount is that current technology cannot reliably detect gluten that is in smaller quantities than this. What that means for you and me is that some foods may still contain trace amounts of gluten, and, depending on the grain and how we react individually, we could still have a reaction to something that claims to be gluten free.

I believe that is what is happening with the pistachios. They probably manufacture these on the same line as a wheat product and cross contamination is occurring. Or, there is an ingredient for flavor that has trace amounts of gluten. At least, this is what I hope is happening. The alternative is that the manufacturer is not labeling the product correctly.

The FDA has mandated that any product that is labeled gluten free must meet the 20 ppm guideline. However, just to add a little confusion, labeling an item gluten free is entirely voluntary. The regulation states that "if" a manufacturer chooses to label an item gluten free, then they "must" follow the 20 ppm guideline. But they are *not* required to label the food if it does in fact contain gluten.

So, what this translates to, is that by law if a manufacturer labels an item gluten free, then it must contain less than 20 ppm of gluten. If a manufacturer does not label a product, then it could, or it could not, contain gluten. Many products that are naturally gluten free, like bottled water, fruits, vegetables, and eggs, will not contain a gluten free label. So if you are interested in a product that is not labeled as gluten free, then you must determine your risk by reading the ingredients, visiting the manufacturer's website, or contacting the manufacturer directly.

The United States Food and Drug Administration also has mandated that labels must contain a listing of the eight main food allergies if present[viii]. These are: milk, egg, fish, crustacean shellfish, tree nuts, wheat, peanuts, and soybeans. The regular ingredient listing, as well as the allergen listing, must list the ingredients in order by weight. So the ingredient that contributes the most weight is listed first, and the ingredient that contributes the least by weight is listed last.

One last point about labeling is that the Food and Drug Administration does not regulate meat, poultry, and some egg products. These are regulated by the US

Department of Agriculture, and therefore, do not fall under the gluten regulation. Also, and much more important to know, is that most alcoholic beverages are regulated by the US Alcohol and Tobacco Tax and Trade Bureau. So alcohol does not abide by the FDA guidelines, although the Alcohol and Tobacco Tax and Trade Bureau does have a similar guideline for voluntary labeling of gluten free[ix].

Many beers and other alcoholic beverages are wheat based. So this is yet one more thing that many gluten intolerant people may have difficulty giving up.

In the end, because of the trace amount issue, many foods might be problematic based on your gluten sensitivity threshold, even if they are labeled gluten free. For me, I am willing to try anything that is arguably gluten free according to labels and manufacturer information. If I become sick, then it becomes a choice to eat or not to eat. For myself, the migraines are the worst choice, so you can bet I won't ever be eating those pistachios again.

Pistachios are not the only food that I have had this issue with. What I discovered is that when I became sick and I could pinpoint it to something that I "hoped" was gluten free, I would not use the best judgement or logic. The idea of losing favorite foods is a difficult prospect, and I would always give the food the benefit of the doubt. I usually paid dearly for this flawed reasoning. Now, I am much better logically, and I have much better self-control.

However, occasionally, I still slip into the illogical John to try and keep a questionable food item on my "to buy" list.

Supermarkets

When it comes to shopping, there are a few supermarkets that really make it easy. They actually have "Gluten Free" tags on the shelves directly below the food items that are gluten free. If I am looking for something in particular, like Progresso soups that are gluten free, then it makes my shopping experience much more expedient and pleasurable. I just scan the shelves by the price stickers and quickly find the gluten free soups. Then I can make my choices and move on much more quickly.

One thing you will want to be aware of, is that although this method is fantastic for the gluten free shopper, just like every other process or procedure, it is not fool proof. On more than one occasion I have purchased a product that contains gluten. But not because the sticker was wrong at the supermarket. The problem is that when the workers stock the shelves, sometimes they have a little more stock, and a little less shelf space, than they planned on. So if they have extra stock with gluten products, then they just put them in the space that has the gluten free sticker.

I am pleased to say that I have never eaten any of these, because I have a habit of reading the labels before I cook at home. On one occasion, from the frozen foods section, I bought a shepherd's pie using the gluten free sticker on the shelf, and it looked delicious (delicious from my gluten free perspective☺). I did not check the label at the store. When I went to cook it, I read the label and discovered the very first ingredient was wheat flour. I brought it back to the store, and they easily let me return it. What the supermarket doesn't realize, of course, is that had I neglected to read the label, I would have become very sick for a week. It is nice that they make it easy to return items, but I am hoping that in the future a little more consideration and diligence will help to avoid this issue altogether.

This stocking items in the wrong section happened on several different occasions before I finally got into the habit of checking the labels right at the supermarket as I take them off of the shelf. It is a good habit to get into, and I find that the errors occur in the frozen food section much more often than dry foods and soups. However, it has happened to me in all sections, so it is a good idea to always check the labels.

Once in a while, I will get sick from something I eat, and I have difficulty pinpointing the offending food. Unfortunately, what I have to do in this case is note the things that I eat in a diary. A diary can be very useful in instances such as this. When I was at the Migraine Clinic, I kept a diary for months. Unfortunately, my immune system was totally messed up, and my gluten intolerance threshold was right on the edge. So I never could find any correlation to the foods I was eating. Now that I am gluten free, my symptoms are gone completely, and my gluten threshold is very, very low. So now I can easily pinpoint offending food over time if I keep a diary.

I discovered that I cannot eat M&Ms with peanuts using this method. Because there is evidently very little gluten in the candy, so it would take a fairly long time for my symptoms to manifest. This caused me to not associate the issue with the candy. Although I do not think that there is gluten directly as an ingredient, I believe that there is cross contamination on the processing lines. I can eat M&Ms without peanuts with no problems. I went on the manufacturer's website, and I discovered that M&Ms are listed in their gluten free section, but the M&Ms with peanuts are not.

So yet another learning experience. Although most candy is gluten free, there are some candies that do have cross contamination because they are processed on the same lines that process wheat products, or they actually do have gluten as an ingredient.

For instance, I loved Lindt chocolates before I became gluten aware. After I knew of my gluten intolerance, I still ate them because I had heard that candy was gluten free. After getting sick a few times, I came to believe it was the chocolates. The next time I went to the chocolate store, I noticed that one of the ingredients is barley malt, which of course contains gluten. After discussing my condition with the store clerk and reading some ingredients, I found out that some of the truffles are gluten free (but very few), and most of the dark chocolate is gluten free. Once I limited myself to these items, I now have no issues.

Potato chips were an educational experience for me as well. Potatoes are gluten free, so potato chips must be gluten free too, right? Not necessarily. It is the same, usual suspects. There can be cross contamination where the chips are processed and/or moved on the same line as wheat products like pretzels. Or they can be flavored with a wheat based coating like barbeque or sour cream & onion.

I have found regular Lays and Frito's Corn Chips to be safe for me, and, through several minor migraine episodes, I discovered that Dorito's Nacho Cheese is not safe. A trip to the manufacturer's websites confirmed this for all three.

The Perspective of Non-Sufferers

It is interesting to note that when I am going through some of these migraine episodes while trying to determine offending foods, the people around me tend to believe that it is something other than gluten. They are in the same state of denial that I was in when I first started becoming gluten free. No one wants to believe that wheat, a staple of the human diet for thousands of years, could possibly be causing a problem.

But I shrug these opinions off, and I stick to my own experiences. Two prime examples are the M&Ms and the Lay's and Dorito's outlined above. My own body, through migraines, lethargy, and digestive discomfort, led me to conclude that M&M's with Peanuts and Dorito's Nacho Cheese had gluten, and that Lay's Regular, Frito's Corn Chips, and M&Ms regular did not contain gluten. After a visit to the manufacturer's websites, my own suspicions were confirmed about which foods contained gluten and which foods did not. Armed with this data, how can I not conclude that my issue is gluten?

When I was living with other people who were not gluten free, I had to keep duplicates of things that I labeled with a marker indicating they were mine and that they were gluten free. For instance, two separate containers of butter. A wheat eating human will butter their wheat bread and toast, and trace amounts and wheat crumbs will remain in the butter.

Wheat bread crumbs = migraine.

So I had my own butter.

But now that I am alone, my home is entirely gluten free. I do not keep gluten containing items for my wheat eating guests. If I have people over for dinner, then I prepare a nice gluten free meal. This helps to minimize and nearly eliminate my chances of eating gluten at home. The only real danger I have now is if I try something new.

Diligence Pays Off

The bottom line for eating gluten free at home is to be diligent, pay attention to your body, and be willing to change your diet to accommodate what your body is telling you. If you are getting sick, keep a diary to help pinpoint the offending food. Always remain open minded and understand that almost any food, because of mass production, can contain gluten.

Try to understand your gluten sensitivity level. I know a few people who are gluten intolerant, and they all have sensitivities that are not as severe as mine. They can "cheat" a little and only pay with a minor upset stomach. I envy them sometimes when I see them chance a few bites of a pastry, because I know that I could never eat even a single bite of that same pastry.

The list of gluten symptoms is long, and we all need to focus on getting our bodies and minds to a point where we have great quality of life. I think I am there right now, and hopefully, with some help from this book, you will be there too.

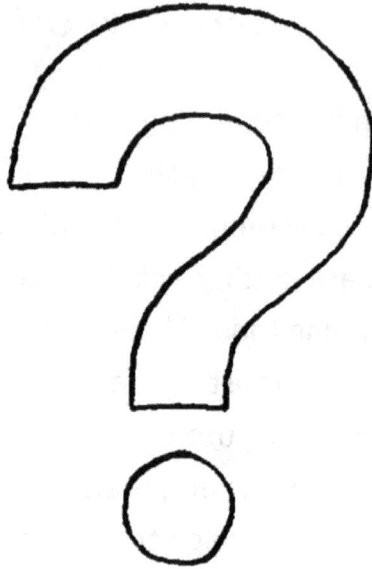

Chapter 6
So What Can You Eat Anyway?

One question I often get is, "So what can you eat anyway?"

When I first started my gluten free dieting, it was extremely difficult. I felt like I couldn't eat anything. It seemed like everything I wanted, I couldn't have. All of the things that my body craved was loaded with gluten.

My experiences have led me to believe that this transitional period is the worst time for someone who is becoming gluten free. My body was used to the gluten, to a certain extent. When I became gluten free, I think my body went into a kind of withdrawal. My body was dependent on the gluten loaded foods. Once I stopped eating them totally, my body craved them. Going to parties, or anywhere for that matter where people were eating, was extremely difficult. In the beginning, I would cheat occasionally, and then pay for it with migraines, lethargy, and vomiting. It literally took me a little longer than a year to be truly gluten free.

I am happy to report that today, the sight or smell of gluten products has absolutely no effect on me. The first year was tough, but relative to my health, my life is better now than it ever was.

Rather than discuss foods that have possibly caused issues for me, (since everyone's level of gluten intolerance is slightly different) I will focus on the foods that I can safely eat. The following list are foods that I eat on a regular basis and that have never resulted in any gluten symptoms for me. Hopefully, in your quest to be gluten intolerant, you can start with this list to give you a head start on "safe" foods. I put safe in quotes because everyone's tolerance is not the same as mine. Hopefully, your tolerance is higher than mine.

Foods that I can personally eat with no gluten related symptoms:

Baking

Bread Crumbs – 4C Gluten Free Crumbs

Brownie Mix – Betty Crocker Gluten Free Chocolate

Brownie Mix – Pillsbury Gluten Free Chocolate Fudge

Cake Mix – Betty Crocker Gluten Free Devil's Food

Cake Mix – Betty Crocker Gluten Free Yellow Cake

Cookie Mix – Betty Crocker Gluten Free Chocolate Chip

Cookie Mix – Betty Crocker Gluten Free Sugar Cookie

Chocolate Chips – Hershey's Milk Chocolate Chips

Chocolate Chips – Hershey's Semi-Sweet Chocolate

Chocolate Chips – Nestle Semi-Sweet Morsels

Chocolate Syrup – Hershey's Syrup

Frosting – Betty Crocker Whipped Butter Cream

Frosting – Betty Crocker Hershey's Milk Chocolate

Frosting – Betty Crocker Rich & Creamy Chocolate

Frosting – Duncan Hines Creamy Classic Chocolate

Frosting – Duncan Hines Creamy Classic Vanilla

Pancake and Baking Mix – Bisquick Gluten Free

Bread and Grains

Bread – Udi's Gluten Free White Sandwich Bread

Bread – Udi's Whole Grain Bread

Cereal – Chex Chocolate, Honey Nut, and Cinnamon

Cereal – Cheerios Chocolate and Regular

English Muffins – Glutino Gluten Free

Candy

Almond Joy Candy Bar

Hershey's Kisses Milk Chocolate

Hershey's Kisses Milk Chocolate with Almonds

Hershey's Kisses Special Dark

Hershey's Milk Chocolate Bar

Hershey's Milk Chocolate Bar with Almonds

Mounds Candy Bar

Reese's Peanut Butter Cups (Regular, not seasonal)

Snickers Bar

Trident Chewing Gum – Tropical Twist

Trident Chewing Gum – Watermelon Twist

Canned, Bottled, and Boxed Goods

Baked Beans – Heinz Home Style Baked Beans Original

Beef Stew – Dinty Moore Beef Stew

Butter Beans – Bush's

Chili – Hormel Chili with Beans

Gravy – Mayacamas Vegetarian Turkey Gravy Mix

Gravy – McCormick Gluten Free Brown Gravy

Gravy – Pioneer Brand Gluten Free Country Gravy Mix

Jelly – Welch's Concord Grape Jelly

Macaroni and Cheese – Annie's Gluten Free

Mashed Potatoes – Idahoan Butter & Herb

Mashed Potatoes – Idahoan Buttery Homestyle

Mashed Potatoes – Idahoan Four Cheese

Mashed Potatoes – Idahoan Sour Cream & Chives

Olives – Pearls Small, Medium, and Large Black Olives

Pasta – Ronzoni Gluten Free Rotini

Pasta – Ronzoni Gluten Free Thin Spaghetti

Peanut Butter – Skippy Creamy

Pickles – Mt. Olive Kosher Dill Spears

Rice – Minute White Rice

Rice – Zatarain's Caribbean Rice Mix

Rice – Zatarain's Dirty Rice Mix

Rice – Zatarain's Jambalaya Mix

Rice – Zatarain's Spanish Rice

Rice – Zatarain's Yellow Rice Mix

Soup – Progresso Chicken & Wild Rice

Soup – Progresso Chicken Cheese Enchilada Flavor

Soup – Progresso Chicken Rice with Vegetables

Soup – Progresso French Onion

Soup – Progresso Garden Vegetable

Soup – Progresso Hearty Black Bean

Soup – Progresso Split Pea with Ham

Spaghetti Sauce – Prego Tomato Basil Garlic

Spaghetti Sauce – Prego Three Cheese

Spaghetti Sauce – Rinaldi Three Cheese

Spaghetti Sauce – Rinaldi Tomato, Garlic & Onion

Taco Shells – Ortega Yellow Corn Taco Shells

Tater Tots – Ore Ida Gluten Free

Tomato Puree - Tuttorosso

Tomatoes, Whole Peeled Plum – Hunt's

Waffle Fries – Ore Ida Gluten Free

Condiments

Barbecue Sauce – Sweet Baby Ray's Honey BBQ Sauce

Ketchup – Heinz Tomato Ketchup

Mayonnaise – Hellmann's Real Mayonnaise

Mustard – French's Classic Yellow Mustard

Picante Sauce, The Original - Pace

Salad Dressing – Wish Bone Light Italian

Salad Dressing – Wish Bone Light Ranch

Salsa – Green Mountain Gringo

Salsa – On The Border Salsa

Soy Sauce – La Choy

Taco Seasoning Mix – McCormick Gluten Free

Teriyaki Stir Fry – La Choy

Dairy

Butter – Land O Lakes Whipped Butter

Cheese – Cabot Extra Sharp and Seriously Sharp

Evaporated Lowfat 2% Milk - Carnation

Ice Cream – Breyers Black Raspberry Chocolate

Ice Cream – Breyers Cherry Vanilla

Ice Cream – Breyers Chocolate

Ice Cream – Breyers Mint Chocolate Chip

Ice Cream – Breyers Natural Strawberry

Ice Cream – Breyers Natural Vanilla

Ice Cream – Breyers Vanilla, Chocolate, Strawberry

Margarine – Land O Lakes Margarine

Milk – Hood 1%
Sour Cream – Tofutti Sour Supreme
String Cheese – Cabot Sharp Light

Fruit
All fresh fruit is naturally gluten free.

Meat
All meat is naturally gluten free. The only caveat is that if there are sauces, breading, or fillers, then you will have to check to be sure they are gluten free.

Bacon – Black Label Maple Bacon
Beef Kielbasa – Hillshire Farms Beef Polska Kielbasa
Cold Cuts - Boar's Head Deli meat and cold cuts
Haddock – Gorton's Grilled Haddock
Sausage – Jones All Natural Fully Cooked Sausage

Snacks
Almonds – Blue Diamond Roasted
Cookies – Glutino Chocolate Chip
Cookies – Glutino Chocolate Vanilla Crème
Cookies – Glutino Vanilla Crème
Corn Chips – Frito's Corn Chips
Corn Chips – Tostito's Original Restaurant Style
Crackers – Milton's Gluten Free Cheddar Cheese
Hot Fudge – Mrs. Richardson's

Nacho Cheese Sauce – Mrs. Renfro's Ghost Pepper

Peanuts – Hampton Farms (In shell)

Popcorn – Pop Weaver Microwave Popcorn

Potato Chips – Lay's Regular

Potato Chips – Utz Honey BBQ, Sour Cream & Onion

Pretzels – Snyder's Gluten Free Prestzels

Vegetables

All vegetables are naturally gluten free. The only caveat is that if there are sauces, breading, or fillers, then you will have to check to be sure they are gluten free.

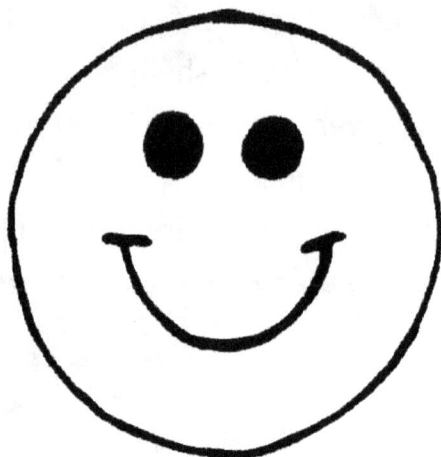

Chapter 7
Last Word

I was inspired to write this book because I found myself recounting my gluten free quest over and over again. Every time I go out to a restaurant with someone new, and they hear my gluten free questions and concerns, they immediately start asking questions. As I recount my years of trials and tribulations, I can see that they are genuinely interested and entertained by my personal experiences.

I hope that my story, especially my mistakes and insights, can serve to help people who are experiencing the same types of symptoms and problems that I have experienced. My goal is to inform some unfortunate souls who, right now, are going through what I went through for over thirty years. My hope is that they will read this and change their habits and thus drastically increase their quality of life.

Gluten is an insidious protein. It can cause many, many health issues. I am positive that there are many more symptoms than what I have listed. Just looking at the broad scope of symptoms, and the seemingly unrelated body areas and functions, makes it clear that gluten can wreak havoc on the entire body in one form or another.

My personal symptoms have disappeared with my change to a gluten free diet. I still have relapses of symptoms due to accidental ingestion of gluten, but overall my quality of life has increased an unbelievable amount.

Being gluten free can be difficult. Manufacturers are now seeing the profitability of offering gluten free products, and they are adding more every day. Flour mixtures are being experimented with that are getting the gluten free products closer in consistency to wheat based products, but unfortunately, there is still a way to go.

The main thing to walk away with after reading this book, is that if you want to be gluten free for medical reasons, or simply to eat healthier, then you must be diligent. Always pay attention to labels. Contact manufacturer websites. Contact manufacturers directly by phone or email. But the single most important thing is to pay attention to your body. Your body has its way of letting you know that something is not right. If your body can't handle gluten, then your body will let you know through headaches, lethargy, IBS, rashes, and many, many other ways. Listen to your body! Hopefully, in the end, just as I did, you will get your body to tell you that everything is ok.☺

References

[i] Staff. (n.d.). *What's wrong with modern wheat?* Retrieved from Grainstorm Heritage Baking: http://www.grainstorm.com/pages/modern-wheat

[ii] *Topomax.* (n.d.). Retrieved from Topomax: http://www.topamax.com/

[iii] Staff, M. C. (n.d.). *http://www.mayoclinic.org/diseases-conditions/migraine-headache/symptoms-causes/dxc-20202434.* Retrieved from http://www.mayoclinic.org.

[iv] *Depakote.* (n.d.). Retrieved from Depakote: https://www.depakote.com/

[v] *Zomig.* (n.d.). Retrieved from Zomig: http://zomig.com/

[vi] Dr. Neal Barnard, D. O. (n.d.). *Sneak Peek: What is Gluten?* Retrieved from The Dr. Oz Show: http://www.doctoroz.com/videos/sneak-peek-what-gluten

[vii] FDA. (n.d.). *Gluten and Food Labeling.* Retrieved from US Food and Drug Administration: http://www.fda.gov/Food/ResourcesForYou/Consumers/ucm367654.htm

[viii] FDA. (n.d.). *Guidance for Industry: A Food Labeling Guide.* Retrieved from US Food and Drug Administration: http://www.fda.gov/Food/GuidanceRegulation/GuidanceDocumentsRegulatoryInformation/LabelingNutrition/ucm064880.htm#label

[ix] TTB. (n.d.). *TTB Rulings.* Retrieved from Alcohol and Tobacco Tax and

Trade Bureau: www.ttb.gov/rulings

www.ingramcontent.com/pod-product-compliance
Lightning Source LLC
Chambersburg PA
CBHW071339290326
41933CB00040B/1698